What international fans are saying about The Bum Gun...

"Bum Gun install - quick and easy"

The Bum Gun was quick and easy to install. What a life changer it is. I can't believe I've been so long without one. How have we missed the boat here in the USA with our penchant for cleanliness? Gone are the days of wiping and obviously still not being really clean.

Rhonda Lackmann - San Jose, California

"One More Female Fan of The Bum Gun Bidet Sprayer"

At first I was apprehensive about buying online, but I got a lot of confidence by the professional approach I received. He was genuinely kind and professional from the start. He recommended the stainless steel Titan model. I installed it myself following the short video he sent. I love my Bum Gun. For any female you cannot live without this amazing invention!! Awesome does not describe it enough.

Hanna Williams, Sri Lanka

The Bum Gun - Cracking piece of kit!

The Bum Gun is an awesome bathroom tool kit! Never thought I'd like the idea but after using it now for 3 years I'd be lost without it. The bum gun really does clean up and refresh the parts other products cannot reach...! The Bum Gun is the most hygienic bathroom tool going!

Paul, Harrogate, N. Yorks, UK

"The Toilet Paper Emancipation Project"

The Bum Gun is a wonderful, high-quality product that'll make you wonder why you ever thought toilet paper was a clean habit! I love being able to use fewer resources. If you want to shrink your environmental footprint, feel cleaner and save money, this is a great way to do it.

Kirsten USA

Essential for dating & marital hygiene

Toilet paper is a barbaric western concept that merely smears the detritus around. It's like giving your nether region a shower after each session, and I guarantee you'll be telling friends & lovers about it. It's the 21st century, and about time that western hygiene caught up. If you're a guy, the girls gossip a lot about foul-smelling men. Using this product ensures you won't be gossip fodder.

Geoff – Cheyenne, WY, USA

Love this product. Wish I had bought one years ago.

Saves a fortune on toilet paper and you feel really clean after. Takes a few days to get used to it but once you get the hang of it, it works a treat.

J. Fay, Newcastle upon Tyne, UK

"Not only a Bidet Sprayer but much much more...."

We have 5 Bum Guns and our customers love them. Money well spent and our customers' bums cleaner.

Paolo, Mamma Mia Italian Restaurant

31 Shocking Health Misconceptions About The Bum Gun

The Smartest Approach To Transform

The Quality of Your Life

Greg Noland

www.thebumgun.com

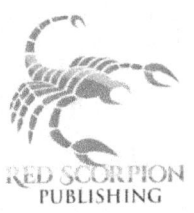

RED SCORPION
PUBLISHING

31 Shocking Health Misconceptions About The Bum Gun

The Smartest Approach To Transform The Quality of Your Life

Copyright ©2016 The Bum Gun Ltd

All trademarks are the property of The Bum Gun Ltd.

Second Edition

ISBN 1537597280
Published by Red Scorpion Marketing & Publishing Ltd

22 Bentinck Lane, East Lane, Hull, East Riding of Yorkshire, HU11 5QR

www.thebumgun.com / www.thebumgun.com/store

"The Biggest Development in Bathroom Hygiene Since Thomas Crapper's 'Bottom Slapper' in 1878"

Contents

"147 Ways To Improve Your Life That Everyone Should Know"

If you are interested in getting your hands on the next book in this series for FREE please email me on: info@thebumgun.com

Use the subject line "Send me my free copy of 147 Ways.." and I'll rush it over to you.

The Bum Gun Irresistible Offer:

Give The Bum Gun Bidet Sprayer a test run today. You Will NEVER regret it… That's a Promise!

www.thebumgun.com/irresistibleoffer-a

Introduction

Hi, hello and G'day

Oh the times, they are a changing!

I want to get straight into this introduction because it's kind of stressing me out.

I've been writing and rewriting this introduction for days. Whatever I come up with just doesn't seem to show the importance of what I'm going to help you discover today. It makes me feel I'm doing a disservice to you, and by doing so could potentially restrict you from discovering the importance of this crucial life changing device.

So please accept my apologies where they are due. But please read until the end of this report because what you're about to learn is worth its weight in gold.

I promise not to take up too much of your time and if you stick with me you'll be glad you did. This whole report is vital to you, but if this introduction doesn't grab your attention then you'll miss this opportunity to transform your life.

I just feel the introduction to this report is just too important to get wrong. I essentially have a huge responsibility to get this right for you.

So let's crack on together. We can't get away from the fact that our lives are more and more affected by poor health choices and a rapidly changing world.

To give you an example, a United States Senate report recently showed us that we're malnourished no matter how much food we eat because our food does not contain the nutrients it should.

This is bad news to learn from our leading authorities that 90% of American people are deficient in these minerals. Also, that a marked deficiency in any one of these important minerals could actually result in disease.

Did you know that spinach, so often thought of as a 'super food' is far from the super provider it once was?

In 1940 – it had 158mgm of iron

In 1965 – it had 27 mgm

Today – it has mere 2.2mgm

So how can facts like this affect your health?

Also, bear in mind cancer is the number 2 killer in the United States. It's a leading cause of death for women aged between 40 and 55.

In 1940 – 1 in 20 women were at risk of breast cancer

Today – 1 in 8 women are at risk

In addition, the National Cancer Institute reports a 126% increase in prostate cancer among men in the last few decades alone. Worrying is that this number is increasing by 1% a year, and currently there are 1.7 million new cases every year.

I think you'll agree that being concerned about our health and nutrition has never been more important.

Alternatively, you might think I'm being over dramatic at this point, over sensational. But look, I know how important this is to you, to humanity and to the environment. There are not many inventions in a single person's lifetime which truly have the potential to shatter the status quo and have the ability to transform the quality of life for so many people.

You might also think 'humanity' is another stab at being dramatic. But I'd appreciate the opportunity to show you by the end of this short report how important this is to your own life.

Why Are We Talking About Poop?

Let's talk crap. Whoops, there I said it. O.K i know it's a bit of a taboo subject, but you've got to admit there have been times when you must have wondered why we are all forced to wipe our private parts continually until we think we are clean (and basically smear) instead of using water to wash our most delicate bits properly.

"Did you know there is at least 0.1 gram of faecal matter in the average pair of underwear of a toilet paper user?"

If you think 0.1 grams doesn't seem like much, do you realise that would equate to 100 million E. coli bacteria floating around in your washing machine? If you're washing five pairs of underpants, then make that 500 million E. coli bacteria floating around among your blouses, and handkerchiefs.

I feel that I was blessed to find The Bum Gun so young. In fact I've been using The Bum Gun for longer than toilet paper right now.

There must also have been times when the abrasive nature of toilet paper has given you unnecessary pain. I know it hurts me every time I'm forced to use it, usually when I'm travelling of course. So much so, that it actually breaks my skin, and results in bleeding. There's just no need for this unnecessary pain and discomfort.

These two points alone should have helped you start thinking of an alternative to toilet paper. But if for a strange reason I haven't won you over just yet how about the repetitive cost of toilet paper, and the hassle of having to remember to buy it every week? This has surely been a hassle you'd rather do without, right? I'm pretty sure you don't like having to fork out for this product every week. It would be better to wipe this product off your weekly shopping list or at least reduce it to once every month or two, right?

In this report I want to provide some clear, honest, answers to some of the misconceptions and misunderstandings about The Bum Gun bidet sprayer.

Is Our World Sustainable?

You'd have to be a Buddhist monk, locked away alone in a cave in the hills of Tibet for the last 30 years to not be aware of the struggles we all face with a rapidly expanding global population and dwindling resources.

Have you ever thought about how many people are using toilet paper in our world? If the current population of the world is 7.4 billion, do you think it is fair to say at least 50% is using toilet paper?

The largest tissue maker in the world, Kimberly-Clark estimates that 1.3 billion people use its tissues every day. That would take a massive amount of resources to supply this demand.

However, for the purpose of this report I would like to focus on the 500 million toilet paper users in the United States, the UK, Australia, Canada and New Zealand.

Why did I choose these countries? Well, these are English speaking countries, and the countries I have done the most research on and the majority are still using toilet paper.

When you consider all the people in the world who have to be supplied with toilet paper each and every day, 500 million is a small portion of the overall figure.

However, what's even more alarming is what will the population of the world be in 2026? – 8.4 billion maybe? How about in 2036? The population of our world, and one which already has limited resources, will probably pass 9 billion by 2036, and more than likely pass 10 billion by 2050.

This is all within our lifetime. I know I'll still be around when 2050 comes around. How about you?

Can we keep ripping out millions of trees every year to satisfy this demand for toilet paper, or find better alternatives?

These are impossible numbers to imagine if we don't start thinking about some really smart alternatives to the way we have been living our lives. If we can do that, then we might be able to sustain these increases in population numbers. However, hitting 8, 9 and 10 billion will create immense problems if we just carry on making the same mistakes with our resources.

So What About The Environmental Footprint of Toilet Paper?

I don't know about you, but I've never been a fan of toilet paper. And I think the vast majority of the English speaking western world would say the same if they thought about it properly.

It doesn't get us properly clean. It can hurt like hell. It costs a lot, especially when you add up the costs over a year for a family. In addition, toilet paper has a huge environmental footprint.

'World Watch' advise us that around 27,000 trees are slain every day to produce toilet paper. The result is that forests worldwide are under assault by the huge toilet paper corporations to fill consumer demand.

It's no secret that, environmentally speaking, many logging companies are far from responsibly managed. The Food and

Agriculture Organization (FAO) of the United Nations, which monitors the state of the world's forests, reports that 13 million hectares of global forests are lost every year.

This can't go on year after year. This includes 6 million hectares of some of the most biologically diverse ecological systems in the world. These numbers aren't tiny blips and I bet you're tired of seeing our beautiful world hammered into the ground just as much as I am.

Bear in mind, this isn't just happening in the Amazon but as published in Trends in Ecology and Evolution, there is an escalating threat to boreal forests in Russia, Alaska, Canada, and Scandinavia. According to the online magazine World Science, the boreal, or northern forest, comprises about one-third of the world's forested area and one-third of the world's stored carbon.

And that's not all, the NGO Forest Ethics reports that "Canada's boreal forest stores 23% of the planet's terrestrial carbon. This is more carbon per acre than any other ecosystem on earth. However, Canada's old growth and intact forests are logged at a rate of five acres a minute, 24 hours a day."

Is The Bum Gun The Perfect Product?

I don't believe that there has ever been a 'perfect product' developed and manufactured in history.

But if I am totally honest, and that's the only way I ever want to be with you, the concept behind The Bum Gun is perfect. Until someone invents a better way to clean than using water, nothing can beat the logic of The Bum Gun.

It gets even better. This simple solution to a common problem also boosts your love-life. If that seems too hard to believe, consider this.

A study conducted in Oxfordshire, England by Dr. J.A. Cameron in 1964 surveyed the underwear of 940 men and found faecal contamination in nearly all of them that ranged from "wasp-coloured" stains to "Mammoth Route 66 skid-marks." Ah, yikes – far too much information!

I'm sorry but I can't mention about the women's drawers!!

The Bum Gun is easy to install, it's cheap to purchase, it's fairly simple in design, and it's ultra-simple to use.

But like I said, nothing is perfect, and in this report you will discover some of its limitations.

If you have a product that you think is perfect, tell me about it – contact me on info@thebumgun.com and I promise I'll mention you in the next edition of this report.

Common Misconceptions and Misunderstandings

The purpose of this report is to address many of the misconceptions and misunderstandings a lot of people have about The Bum Gun and bidet sprayer technology.

I will also try to address some of the flaws The Bum Gun may have in an open, honest and transparent way.

But look, the truth is ever since I discovered The Bum Gun I've never ever wanted to return to toilet paper. When I travel it's always a really big concern about having to use toilet paper. Since using The Bum Gun I also have never taken a day off work sick. This is going back to 1991. How about you? How many days have you taken off in the last 20 years?

I can't say 100% that only The Bum Gun can take credit for my healthy state but I know it's got a lot to do with it.

These days I am able to work 18 hour days when I want to and still hit the gym 4 or 5 times a week.

I see far too many people these days drained of all energy and constantly worrying about what the future holds for them. It's no wonder, considering all the obstacles in most people's lives.

There's no doubt in my mind that The Bum Gun can bring some comfort, peace and pleasure to your life.

Now, I know what you're thinking... I would say that to sell the product.

Yes, I'd like to make money to take care of my family and my loved ones.

However, my main goal here is to make a difference in our world. I also aim to help as many people as possible and make my family proud for generations that I actually gave something back to our society.

Look, it's quite simple. If you find nothing wrong with toilet paper, perhaps I will never win you over. That's your loss my friend. I know that's pretty blunt, but I'm a straight-to-the-point kinda person. And that's exactly what you can expect from The Bum Gun too. No fluff, just results.

And besides, does it really matter if I make a bit of money? Especially since you will see a return on your investment (ROI) within 2 to 4 months?

The bottom line is, The Bum Gun will not only save you a lot of pain and discomfort but could also save you a ton of money on toilet paper and the costs going to buy it but also prevent months of potential lost income for you and your family before you all retire. Isn't that a huge advantage to you?

I've Never Even Heard of The Bum Gun!

If you have never even heard of The Bum Gun before, hey, look it isn't your fault. All this information might be coming down on you like a ton of bricks. But please have patience and keep reading. The Bum Gun is a completely new product to the west, and I would say the vast majority of those reading this report, never grew up with The Bum Gun installed in their bathroom.

But I know one thing is certain, by the time you finish reading this short report, I'll have opened your eyes about The Bum Gun and also helped you become aware that there is an alternative to toilet paper. You'll also realize that you no longer have to be restricted by toilet paper anymore.

You and your loved ones actually do have a much cleaner, more comfortable, cost saving device....waiting to serve you.

There are bound to be a certain number of misunderstandings about this device.

So shall we get started covering some of them?

31 Dangerous Health Misconceptions

Here are 31 of the most common misconceptions I've found people have with The Bum Gun. These have been collected over the last three years. These comments are usually the first hurdle before people are confident to try The Bum Gun for themselves. Be careful, once reading this report I bet you won't want to return to toilet paper again.

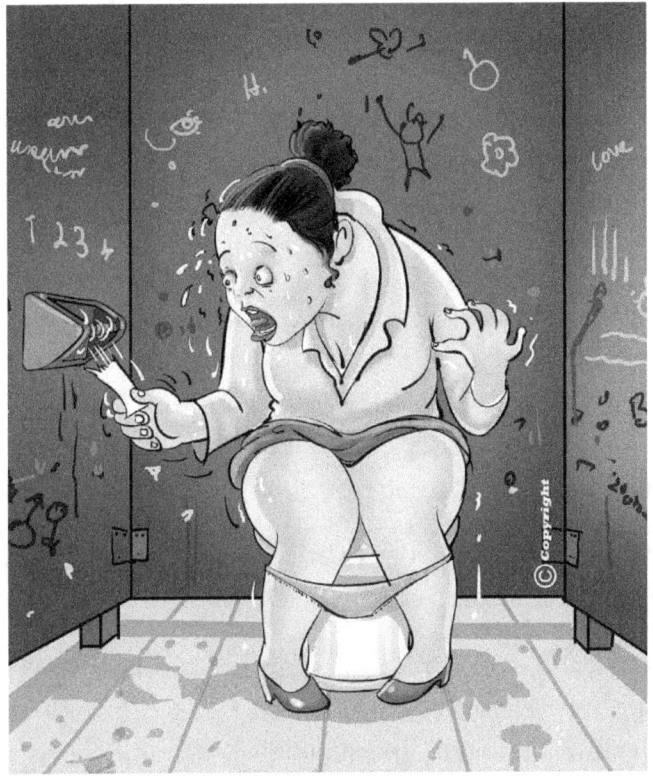

1. The Bum Gun wastes water

I started this report with this one because it is one of the biggest fallacies about The Bum Gun, and one that really needs explaining. Yes, The Bum Gun Uses Water. There are some people on the internet who say that Bum Guns wastes water.

Obviously, there is an amount of water used every time you use The Bum Gun. However, the amount of water used is minimal when compared with the millions of gallons of water used to produce toilet paper every year. In my studies, The Bum Gun uses about 150-250 ml of water with every use, so perhaps 1.0 to 1.5 litres per day. The average toilet, even the economical flushing toilets use about 1.6 gallons per flush. In my book 'The Book on The Bum Gun' I go into an intensive detail about how much water The Bum Gun saves over toilet paper, especially when other changes in toilet habits are adopted when making the switch to The Bum Gun.

Also, we use water to wash every other part of our bodies so why would we restrict ourselves a little water to clean our most private parts? A no brainer when you think about it.

A little bit of information for you, let's call it useful trivia if you're concerned that The Bum Gun will increase your water usage. Try flushing your toilet less. You might have heard the term "If it's yellow, let it mellow. If it's brown, flush it down". I've followed this principle for years now, and have saved thousands of gallons of water over the years.

Even if you only flushed your toilet once less per day, your water use from The Bum Gun would equal out.

The National Geographic claims about 26 billion gallons of water are used each day in the United States, of which about 6 billion gallons is used to operate toilets.

The size of toilet tanks vary, but let's say yours is 1.6 gallons. If you only flushed one time less per day, that would be a saving of over 584 gallons. If you flushed 2 times less per day that would save 1,168 gallons over a year.

Remember, that is only talking about how much you could save. How much could your whole family save over a year if you tried this new approach? How about if 50 million people in a country flushed only one time less per day. This would save an astronomical amount of water.

I would also like to add, it wouldn't take much effort to flush two or three times less per day.

More Ideas to Save Water

Fix leaks. Toilet leaks can cost you up to 200 gallons of water each day, the same amount it would take to wash 10 loads of clothes in an Energy Star-rated washing machine.

Keep it clean: Don't use your toilet as a trash can. Toss dead bugs and tissues into the compost pile or trash. Extra junk in your wastewater means more energy spent to clean it at the sewage treatment plant.

Install a dual flush toilet: or if you can't afford to replace your toilet I've heard some people put a large house brick in the tank to reduce how much water fills into the tank

2. Why is it so important that I clean myself so much down there? I've got by for years with toilet paper. I don't get what the big hoo-ha is about these Bum Guns.

Ok, if this is your train of thought on the matter, then perhaps I will never win you over. But what about your family members? The Bum Gun will improve your family's quality of life even if you're not interested. Just because you wish to struggle on with toilet paper, does that mean your family members have to do without also? If you have children, they deserve to have access to the best advancements in technology for the benefit of their personal hygiene and quality of life.

If you have a teenage daughter, are you aware that the average female teenage girl uses more than ten times the amount of toilet paper than other members of the household? The reason being they are struggling to feel clean and pure with just toilet paper.

3. Washing your face is more important than washing your privates. I don't think I need The Bum Gun.

Much like no.2 above, if washing your private parts is not important to you, then what about the discomfort of using abrasive toilet paper on your private parts? In my opinion, proper cleaning of your sensitive intimate areas is just as important as washing your face, perhaps even more so! I agree that when we don't wash our face, dirt, germs and other impurities that remain can cause skin problems. But likewise, improper cleaning of your private parts is neglecting proper personal care that can result in much more serious complaints and diseases.

4. Do you truly believe the Bum Gun option is cleaner and healthier?

The Bum Gun really is the hottest modern development in personal hygiene for years.

If you are asking yourself "Do I really need The Bum Gun?" I think what I've been saying for years and what I heard Dr. Oz say on the Oprah show recently strikes the truest cord possible - "If you had pee or poop on your hand, you wouldn't wipe it off with toilet paper, would you? You'd wash it off, right?" The Bum Gun gives you the technology to do that in the most efficient and comfortable way possible.

I was again reminded of this fact this morning, when I was washing my car. There were some particularly grimey splodges of bird poo on my windows that had crusted over. As I scrubbed at these monstrosities, I realized I was using water, and not a wad of tissue to wipe them off. Roughly the same deal, wouldn't you agree?

5. Isn't The Bum Gun difficult to install?

While installing a stand-alone bidet will require quite a lot of plumbing experience to install, one of the huge benefits of The Bum Gun installation is that there is very little to it. To install The Bum Gun you don't need to be concerned with any electrics such as for the Japanese toilet seats. Just follow the simple instructions in one of the videos below and in no time flat, you'll have your very own Bum Gun fully operational (sorry if we don't have your preferred language yet). The install process requires nothing more than what you would find in a normal tool box and works with your existing system.

Please see our installation videos on YouTube for clear instructions.

6. I don't want to alter my plumbing to install The Bum Gun.

The Bum Gun works well with your existing plumbing, as you can see in the videos above. In most cases there is no need for additional modifications that need to be made to your existing set up. However, in the eventuality a plumber is required to modify your existing setup, it will be an extremely small price to pay for the numerous benefits for you and all the family once installation is complete.

7. I read on your website that your fittings are all half inch. I live in an area that doesn't have half inch piping, so how will your Bum Guns connect to my plumbing?

Yes, our thread sizes are standard 1/2 inch BSP thread sizes. In some cases, not all, in the USA there are different thread sizes of the feed pipe coming out of the wall. To convert this thread size for The Bum Gun is simple. All that is required is a simple connection convertor. These can be found in any local hardware store. We can also provide technical drawings for any customer who needs more information, just get in touch. In my experience all thread sizes in the UK, Canada and Australia, and most parts of the USA are 1/2 inch BSP.

8. Water and electricity doesn't seem right to me. Plus I think The Bum Gun wastes electricity so this would prevent me using one.

Yes, electricity and water is a bad mixture. However, there is no electricity required to use The Bum Gun. You may be confused by the Japanese bidet toilet seats which have a dryer which requires the electrical source.

9. I've heard Bum Guns leak and I'll end up with a flooded bathroom.

Yes, there have been cases of cheap bidet sprayers malfunctioning. This is why our bidet sprayers are made of stainless steel and also come with high pressure stainless steel spiral hoses as standard.

I would advise you stay away from cheap copy bidet sprayers you might find on places like eBay and Amazon with plastic connectors, PVC hoses, inferior plastic sprayer handles and trigger mechanisms. One important first step to check when buying a bidet sprayer is whether they offer a 5 year warranty.

I also recommend every Bum Gun is fitted with one of our stainless steel isolating safety valves for even more protection and peace of mind.

Also, the stainless steel isolating safety valves double up in use by reducing the high water pressure in some countries to prevent your private parts ending up on the bathroom mirror.

Yikes, wouldn't want that, would we?

10. I've heard Bum Guns from China leak. I have a carpeted bathroom, so I don't want to end up with a soggy carpet.

As mentioned in no.9 above, there are varieties of quality in the design and construction of bidet sprayers just like any product. When buying your own bidet sprayer I would advise to make sure it is made from stainless steel or at least brass. And also come with a 5 year warranty.

11. This invention might be ok in Thailand where all you have to do is use the bum gun and spray down the entire bathroom and it all drains out. But in a western bathroom you can't just spray down with water cause there's no place for it to drain.

Yes, The Bum Gun does have a variety of uses and one of them is the ability to quickly, efficiently and easily rinse down the entire bathroom. As most Thai bathrooms are designed as wet rooms, this is possible. However, with the majority of UK houses for example, with floorboards and often carpet, this would obviously not be possible.

But bathroom cleaning is only one extra benefit of The Bum Gun. You can read all about the benefits of The Bum Gun in my report *'147 Ways To Improve Your Life That Everyone Should Know'*.

Carpets in a bathroom? – Yes, some people feel it is really nice to stand on carpet after their shower, while they shave, comb their hair and get dressed.

12. My plumbing mate told me the water pressure in Australia and UK is too powerful for Bum Guns.

As mentioned in point no.9 above, that is what the stainless steel isolating safety valve is for. You can see our safety valves in our installation videos.

13. I've bought some Bum sprayers from eBay before but I wasn't satisfied by the spraying nozzle. Sometimes water seemed to spray out too far.

This is a good point about cheaper bidet sprayers which can be found on places like eBay. They act like "kitchen salad sprayers" where the spray direction needs to cover a wide area. Whereas for cleaning your private parts you need the opposite. You need a very direct, controlled spraying area, such as the size of a large coin. This is another massive benefit of The Bum Gun because we have spent the time to develop our Bum Guns to spray in a very specific manner so you're not soaking a large area of your bottom, just your flower bud.

14. My kids will play with a bumwash sprayer too much, flooding the bathroom.

I honestly can't vouch for everyone's children. Perhaps your kids will be intrigued by their new Bum Gun after the initial installation. However, I very much doubt most kids will have water fights flooding their bathrooms. Asian kids are smart enough to know that would be good reason for a hiding, and I think most western kids are equally smart as their Asian cousins. Plus I've never heard of western families living in Asia complain about their kids running riot in the bathroom with their Bum Guns.

15. I think my children won't be able to learn how to use these toilet hoses.

Similar to point no.14 above, I don't see any difference in intelligence between Asian and western kids. Asian kids learn from a very young age how to clean up after the toilet. Plus western children living in Asia follow suit and learn quickly with no problems. No reason why your kids can't learn quickly too if they're given the chance.

16. I actually bought one of your OMG teen books on Amazon for my teenage daughter because she uses bucket loads of toilet paper every week. Is the Bum Gun only for females?

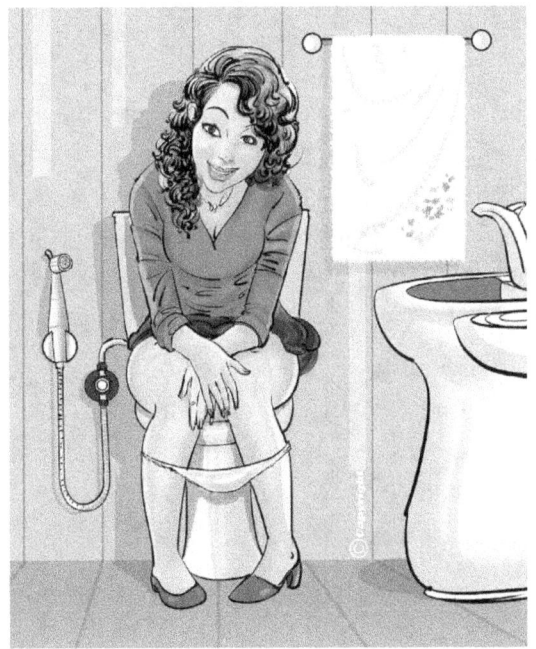

All females are amazed at the functionality of The Bum Gun because they have front and back to wash after toilet visits. But all males benefit massively from getting 'shower fresh clean' after a no.2.

17. In a public bathroom, I don't want to pick up The Bum Gun to find shit all over the end. The end of the hose could be contaminated with bacteria.

In over 20 years using public bathrooms in Asia, I have never seen the end of a bidet sprayer soiled. Could it be possible, I suppose so yes. But that should not deter you from installing The Bum Gun in your own private bathroom. Then it's up to you to use it properly.

18. These toilet hoses might be fine in a tropical country when you can dry your body in seconds, but I don't want to walk around with a wet bum all day and risk getting a rash on my private bits. Toilet paper might not be perfect at cleaning, but at least it gets you dry.

This is always a strange misconception to me, but one that does come up from time to time. After cleaning yourself with The Bum Gun, yes your private parts will be a little wet. But what do you do after a shower? After you've washed your face? You use a towel, right? Same deal with The Bum Gun. What most people do is to keep a flannel sized towel hanging next to their toilet to dry off with. Obviously for public bathrooms, you simply use a few sheets of toilet paper to dry off with. Although some customers tell me they use a handkerchief to dry off with. But one thing's a dead cert, you do NOT end up with water everywhere like some people believe.

19. I live in Canada where the water is freezing cold. I don't want to give myself a shock of a lifetime, and possibly rupture my insides by spraying ice cold water up my clacker!

For customers who require warm water for their Bum Gun, we simply guide them to an appropriate website which has suitable mixers. You will be able to find something very similar in your local hardware store.

This warm water mixer can be used to save your crown jewels if you live in an area with particularly cold water.

20. If the Bum Gun is so good, then why do the North Americans, Brits and Antipodeans prefer toilet paper?

Just because many people are not yet aware of recent developments in personal hygiene technology does not mean, in any way shape or form, that people prefer toilet paper. To support this is the fact that absolutely no one returns to toilet paper after discovering the benefits of The Bum Gun. This statement is SO important I will repeat it for you, just to make sure you understand this fact and are fully able to comprehend what this will mean to you and your family:

"Absolutely no one returns to toilet paper after discovering the benefits of The Bum Gun"

21. Why should I have to fork out $80 when I can buy a pack of perfectly good toilet paper for $7?

Firstly, "perfectly good" toilet paper is definitely a matter of opinion. Perfectly good for what? Cleaning properly like water can? I'm afraid not. Secondly, yes you will have to make a small initial investment to purchase The Bum Gun, and perhaps for installation also. However, you should see a return on investment (ROI) within 2 to 4 months depending on how big your family is, and how much toilet paper you all use. If you have a couple of female teenagers in your family, most likely a lot sooner.

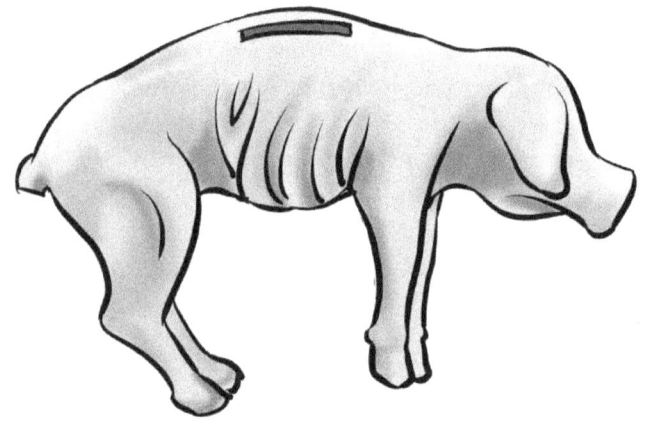

"Don't waste your hard earned money on toilet paper anymore. Save for years with The Bum Gun"

But then for years to come you'll be saving heaps of money by not having to drive to your supermarket every week and keep purchasing toilet paper.

The savings you'll make by not having to buy any or as much toilet paper as usual, might not be enough to buy a car. But in these tough economic times any savings on your total shopping bill are gladly received, right? And why not do your bit to help the environment at the same time?

22. My home is in rural Wales, so we are off the standard water mains. If I don't have enough water pressure at my house, the Bum Gun won't work.

You got me on this one. Yes, The Bum Gun needs water pressure to function. If you live in an area with no water mains pressure, you could benefit from one of our Travel Bidet Sprayers. Please get in touch if this interests you.

23. I've seen bidets and bumguns in hotels I have been at, but I didn't quite know how to use them so I just avoided them. (Looked kind of creepy.)

The Bum Gun is essentially a mini-shower hose, not much different from the one you use to shower with every day. Nothing to be scared about my friend. Simply point in the direction of contact and squeeze the trigger.

24. I don't believe The Bum Gun is more eco-friendly, as you have to ship them half way across the globe, which wastes energy.

Yes, we currently ship our Bum Guns from Thailand to our customers, mostly in the UK, USA, Canada and Australia. Admittedly this is not the preferred situation, but we don't have much choice at the moment. Thais are very experienced and professional with the design and manufacture of this product and to provide all our customers with the highest quality of product this is our chosen setup.

Yes, the distance from factory to customer is far, but at least this is once in 5 years or more. In contrast, toilet paper is shipped across the globe in massive quantities every week of the year. And then transported by truck from large warehouses every week, for you to then drive to when purchasing.

25. Do water companies really prefer bidet sprayers to toilet paper and wet wipes?

While toilet paper at least breaks down fairly quickly, wet wipes most definitely do not. You don't have to try too hard to find information from our water companies complaining of the massive costs of flushing wet wipes down our toilets. These are costs we all have to bare, which is hardly fair.

26. I don't believe wet wipes don't disintegrate when we flush them down the toilet.

If you don't believe me, try searching "Fatbergs" on YouTube for just one source of information.

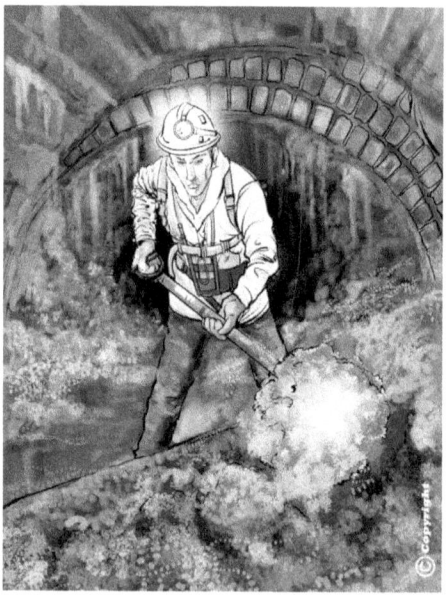

Thames Water in London had to deal with a 15 ton fatberg in London sewers recently. Utility workers spent 6 weeks to dig out this monstrosity after Kingston residents reported not being able to flush their toilets. Gordon Hailwood, waste contracts supervisor for Thames Water, said this was the biggest 'fatberg' in history. So what caused this massive problem?

Lumps of festering food fat mixed with wet wipes caused this serious problem in London's sewers. If they hadn't discovered this fatberg in time, raw sewage could have started spurting out of manholes and into people's homes across the whole of Kingston.

I could go on and on. But the simple fact is London's definitely not the only water company to have to deal with this wet wipes problem.

27. What about water shortages? What happens when these bumguns become mainstream, there will be bitching from some sources about the extra water usage, given the problems we have in Australia.

As mentioned in no.1, we can all save a huge amount of water over a year by flushing the toilet less. How about installing lever taps to your sinks and even the shower? So when you are lathering up you can easily turn off the tap. Over a year, this would save hundreds if not thousands of gallons in your house, especially if you encourage all the family to follow your lead.

I advised my local gym to install lever taps 3 or 4 years ago, and the owner told me this has saved their water usage by almost 30% which I think is fantastic.

How about filling a jug of water and keeping it in the fridge so you don't always have to run the tap when you fancy a cold glass of water?

28. My friend bought a Bum Gun from eBay and he said it didn't even last one year. And, I don't want to buy an Asian product, I want to buy something manufactured in the UK.

As mentioned earlier buying from eBay can be tricky. Please practice due diligence when purchasing your bidet sprayers and also make sure the company selling the products is a fully registered company, and not some fly by night operation. Here today, gone tomorrow.

Needless to say, I would love to be able to set up a factory in the UK to manufacture Bum Guns locally but unfortunately that's impossible right now. Asia is the factory of the world at the moment, and I bet the majority of everyone's house has Asian made products. The Bum Gun is a specialist piece of kit and for now at least I'd say, leave the manufacturing to the professionals.

29. I read somewhere that even your products are not perfect and you had to send a replacement once.

I'll fully admit that even our Bum Guns have had issues in the past. It is my goal to develop the "near perfect" product if I can. But I am a realist and know that there are things that can go wrong with any product. The iPhone is a fantastic invention, but sometimes they go wrong.

I once saw a Rolls Royce being pushed into a closed container. Obviously the Rolls Royce Company doesn't want to show a broken down 'Roller' being carted back for repairs.

The most important thing is the ability and quality of the company and how they react when one of their products doesn't live up to their usual standards.

This is why we offer our customers a 5 year warranty to give them peace of mind when purchasing.

30. I live in Australia so how can I get one of your Bum Guns? Availability, plumbing sizes?

We ship all round the world. Please visit our Online Store at www.thebumgun.com/store to make your purchase. If you would prefer to just send your order in my email, please use:

info@thebumgun.com and I'll answer you as soon as I can. Pipe sizes of our products are half inch BSP which matches Australia.

31. I'm an American and a bum gun fan. Every new house in America has a bum gun, the only problem is that it's mounted on the kitchen sink! How am I supposed to get my ass up there?

I believe that is what is called a "Salad Sprayer" perhaps best not to climb all over your sink my friend. Just get a proper Bum Gun installed and spray "your salad" in the bathroom.

Final Words

There you have it. ***'31 Shocking Health Misconceptions About The Bum Gun'*** that I have come across over the last few years. I hope this has been an informative read and that I have cleared up any concerns or misunderstandings you may have had.

I called them *'dangerous'* because that's what happens with misconceptions if we aren't careful. I don't want someone else's misunderstandings and ignorance of The Bum Gun cloud your judgement and possibly prevent you from benefitting from bidet sprayer technology. We are after all tribal people. It's in our roots, so we follow mostly what everyone else follows.

Obviously I didn't set out to change the whole world with this report. Although I have talked about some huge population numbers and multiple countries, this report is all about you.

Yes, just you and your family members. They are your whole world, right? They are always there for you. And you want the best life possible for them.

By writing this report I hope I have squashed any fears you might have had about test driving The Bum Gun for yourself.

Better yet, if I have succeeded then I hope I'll be hearing from you very soon with your first order. To sweeten the process I've prepared an irresistible offer for you at the end of this report, consisting of two Titan Bum Guns, our best-seller.

I hope you take this opportunity to make a huge step change in your life. If you have two bathrooms then great. If you only have one, then please use the other Bum Gun as a gift for someone very special to you who you think will appreciate this upgrade in their life.

Needless to say, almost anyone who uses the toilet – with the exception perhaps of the guys from the 'What Doesn't Suck' blog (no pleasing everyone) – will be clamouring for this special offer.

Consequently, I can only keep this offer open until my current stocks run out. So don't sit on this offer and end up doing nothing.

Will You Choose To Test Drive The Bum Gun?

Nobody really wants to have to go to the toilet. But anyone in his or her right mind DOES want to avoid the misery of broken skin from abrasive toilet paper, not feeling properly clean, *'itchy-butt-itis'* and having to waste your hard earned money every week, on the nasty old toilet paper.

Enter the 21st century's answer to an age old problem. The Titan Bum Gun bidet sprayer.

Never again will you have to smear around hoping to get clean. The Titan has been designed to provide you a very controlled direct spray action to ensure a 'shower fresh clean' every time and in seconds, without even having to get undressed.

It's up to you now. This is the time for you to take action. So please move to the next page titled **'Irresistible Offer'**, get ready to ***'Transform the Quality of Your Life After Every Bathroom Visit'.***

Go on, go ahead and email me now before you forget and miss this chance altogether.

Irresistible Offer

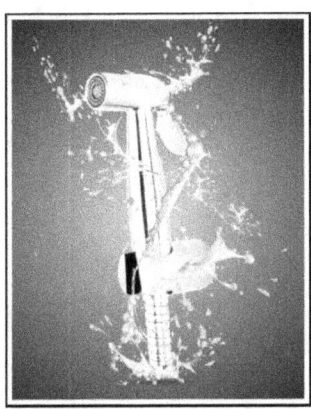

You have spent the time to read through the whole of my report so I would like to make it easy for you to jump on-board and get started with The Bum Gun.

Now to be honest with you, you could decide to go with a Japanese electronic toilet seat. But you could be looking at spending at least $500. That's a bit pricey.

Plus in my experience I don't think these bidet seats are as good as The Bum Gun. Apart from the price, I don't think they give you as much flexibility and control with the direction of your water spray. With The Bum Gun you keep your body still and direct the spraying nozzle. I found that with the electronic seats I had to squirm my body so that the sprayer could reach the desired spot. Plus I have found the jet spray is usually too weak for a proper cleaning. In addition, the 'blow drier' was too weak, and would have needed a few minutes to get dry.

So, to help you get started with The Bum Gun I'm going to make this super easy for you with an irresistible offer.

If you can help me spread the word according to The Bum Gun, then you can make a huge saving today.

In fact, I'm even going to sweeten the deal.

So when you grab two Titan Bum Guns today, you'll receive them for the once in a lifetime low price. You have two options. Option A with the 3 way valves, and Option B without, in case you wish to go with a warm water mixer.

Option A: Two x Titan bidet sprayers and two x 3 way valves for the low price of £150.00

www.thebumgun.com/irresistible-offer-a

Option B: Two x Titan bidet sprayers for the low price of £105.00

www.thebumgun.com/irresistible-offer-b

Notes:

a) Both prices include worldwide shipping by registered mail.
b) Free gifts included with both options.
c) This offer could close at any time, up to my discretion.

But I should warn you this offer will **not** be open for long.

I know that might put a bit of pressure on you, so I'm going to make your decision extremely simple.

You can grab your Titan Bum Guns today, try them out, and if for some reason you don't feel much cleaner than toilet paper, you're covered by our 60 day guarantee.

Because of the limited nature of this offer, I don't want to take up too much more of your time.

Click one of the BUY buttons above or email me right now on info@thebumgun.com with your choice of Option A or B, with your postal address and mobile phone number, and I'll send you an invoice to make payment.

Again, I'm Greg Noland and I'm incredibly excited for you to jump in and get started with your very own Titan Bum Gun bidet sprayers.

Talk to you soon.

Email me now to start changing your family's life forever.

YOU and all your family deserve the best in life, don't you?'

Greg Noland

Dedicated to improving hygiene,

Founder, CEO & Author

The Bum Gun Ltd

www.thebumgun.com

60 Day Trial For The Bum Gun

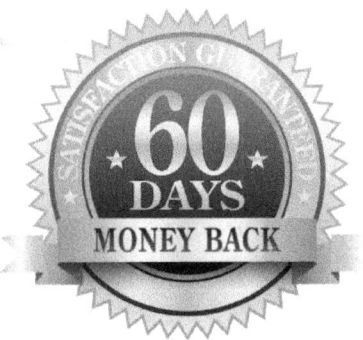

To help make this big change in your life super easy I'd like to give you an offer you can't refuse. I'll give you a clear cut 60 day test period to try The Bum Gun for yourself. If after trying The Bum Gun you honestly feel toilet paper is better than The Bum Gun after two full months of testing, simple return your bidet sprayer to get all your money back. Is that fair?

Heck, you can even keep the free gifts you receive when you order your bidet sprayer as my thank you for giving The Bum Gun a try.

You don't have to deal with toilet paper pain, discomfort, skid stains and nasty gling-ons any longer.

Start enjoying your new life feeling "shower fresh clean" all day long, experience more energy and vigour, and start saving your money today.

Oh, and get ready for your new "rockstar" status when all your family members are thanking you for having the vision to test drive The Bum Gun!!

"Coupled with widespread use of The Bum Gun and better hand hygiene practices will prevent infections, reduce absenteeism and improve performance."

YOU and all your family deserve the best in life, don't you?

So go on, email me now to start changing your family's life forever.

Dedicated to improving hygiene,

Greg Noland

Founder, CEO & Author
The Bum Gun Ltd
www.thebumgun.com

Do You Have a Question?

If you have a question that is not answered below, please email us on info@thebumgun.com and we'd be happy to answer you as soon as possible.

What is The Bum Gun?

The Bum Gun range of hand held bidet sprayers have been designed and manufactured for every man, woman and child on our planet for use instead of toilet paper. The Bum Gun is an important bathroom device that effectively cleans your private parts by spraying an invigorating, cleansing jet of water to this area.

Why do I need The Bum Gun?

I think this is a very common question for anyone who has not had the opportunity to discover The Bum Gun yet. I thought the same. I guess we are all brought up to believe there is no alternative to toilet paper. But as with most things, technology develops. Now in the 21st century this very smart device is here to improve your life, and help you get much cleaner after every toilet visit. You just need to give The Bum Gun 2 or 3 days, and I promise you that you will never go back to toilet paper. That is my iron clad guarantee to you.

Is The Bum Gun for everyone?

The Bum Gun is an ideal product for every home, office, factory, business premises or sports facility and anywhere which has a toilet. The Bum Gun is ideal for everyone who cares about their personal hygiene. The Bum Gun is also perfect for kids, females, the elderly and the physically challenged. Due to The Bum Gun's compact size it is ideal for smaller bathrooms where a standard bidet system struggles to fit in.

Can The Bum Gun help with my hygiene?

Using water has always been the healthier, more comfortable and cleaner option than abrasive toilet paper. When using The Bum Gun every time you use the bathroom you prevent your hands from coming into contact with many germs and bacteria.

Is The Bum Gun hard wearing and durable?

There are varieties of bidet sprayers all over the world, in various degrees of quality. We have chosen the best quality devices we could find. Admittedly, many of the cheaper versions on the market do not have quality, durable components, are not tested rigorously and consequently don't come with extensive warranties like The Bum Gun. Note: Please be careful of the cheap quality bidet sprayers that could crack and leak causing water damage to your bathroom.

What is The Bum Gun made from?

All essential core components, such as the body, hose, collars and trigger are made of premium 304 stainless steel so you never have to worry about cracks and splits causing leaks common with the cheap plastic and PVC copies you might have seen.

Ordering & Making Payments

• Using PayPal: All our products can be purchased immediately through The Bum Gun website using PayPal. If you are not familiar with PayPal, don't worry. It is very simple and secure.
• Note: You can still use your debit or credit card even if you don't have a PayPal account.
• Phone Orders: We can take payment over the telephone.

- You can simply email us your order if you'd prefer.
- We will email you an invoice for all your products.

How long does delivery take?

We promise to do our best to ensure your order is delivered within 5 to 14 days. We use the Registered Mail postal service or a leading   courier service of our choice. We will confirm your order by e-mail. Our products are offered   subject to availability. If we cannot supply you with any product in your order we will contact you by email or phone to advise you and offer an alternative, or refund if preferred. You will be responsible for any taxes or customs duties that may be applicable to your country. In the event a delivery attempt is made and the customer is not available to receive the goods or refuses to accept the goods and they are returned to us the customer will be held responsible for the initial delivery charges and subsequent charges to have the goods re-delivered.

International Bidet Sprayer Orders

If you are not in the UK you can still order our products. Simply email   your   choice   of   products   to   us at info@thebumgun.com with your delivery address and we will reply with your total cost. **Note: There may be import taxes to pay in your country.**

Installation, Use & Maintenance

You can check out our Installation video on YouTube in 3 Languages. The Bum Gun is easy to install, simple to use and environmentally friendly. The Bum Gun attaches to your existing toilet providing the same benefits as the expensive full size bidet system. Do I need to buy any other components to install The Bum Gun? The Bum Gun comes with everything you need to carry out the installation on a standard toilet which has a BSP 1/2″ fitting outlet. The pack includes The Bum Gun, the hose, washers, wall mount, screws and raw plugs.

How long does it take to install The Bum Gun?

A qualified plumber would take someone in the region of 10-20 minutes to install The Bum Gun based on most plumbing configurations. You can check out our Installation video on YouTube in 3 Languages.

How do you control the pressure?

We believe The Bum Gun must be fitted with a "T" joint, or 3 way valve to control the pressure of the sprayer. This way, the toilet's water tank fills quickly and the water pressure to the hand spray is reduced to a lower pressure. Then you use the trigger on The Bum Gun to reach the desired spray pressure. Warning: Do not use The Bum Gun without a "T" joint, or 3 way isolating valve to control the pressure of the sprayer.

Do I really need an Isolating Valve?

We believe The Bum Gun should be fitted with an Isolating Valve and turned off after every use. This ensures maximum safety and relieves the build of possible pressure. Warning: Do not use The Bum Gun without an Isolating Valve to control the pressure of the sprayer.

Tools required for The Bum Gun installation

For most installations, the only tools needed to install The Bum Gun is an adjustable spanner, and a drill and screwdriver to fit the wall bracket. Some plumbers tape is also advisable for a tight leak free seal.

Safety & Non Return Safety Valve

The Bum Gun must be fitted with a non-return safety valve. This valve allows the incoming flow of water from the hose to The Bum Gun. But back flow is prevented thanks to the self-closing valve system so zero un-pure water enters the public water supply system should The Bum Gun be dropped into the toilet bowl by mistake. Warning: However, you should ALWAYS be sat on the toilet whenever using The Bum Gun, and replace carefully and securely into the wall bracket before standing.

Water Regulations

You must carry out the installation of your Bum Gun within your local water regulations. If you are unsure of your legal requirements please ask for advice from a professional plumber. For further details about the U.K. water regulations please contact them directly or visit the Water Regulations Advisory Scheme website at www.wras.co.uk – Or similar water authorities in your country.

About the Author

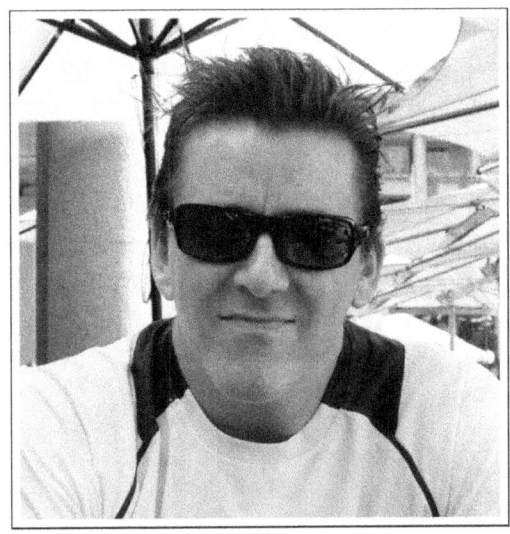

Greg Noland is the CEO & Founder of The Bum Gun Company. He is an entrepreneur, internet marketer, author, life coach, health & fitness enthusiast, and when he can find the time, a world traveller. Greg started his first business at the age of 9, and had a team of 4 employees before his eleventh birthday, and business has just grown since then.

Greg is the author of *The Book On The Bum Gun – The Secrets to The King of Personal Hygiene*, and the co-author with his wife of the *OMG Teen Book Series,* starting with *OMG I'm a Teen! Now What? - A Survival Guide for Teenage Girls. (www.omgteenbookseries.com)*

After surviving a fatal car accident at the age of 29, Greg received what he calls "The Mission to Contribute": a calling to help others get the most out of their lives. Since then, he has dedicated his life to helping people improve the quality of their life with The Bum Gun bidet sprayer.

The 5/20 Plan

Greg's major plan for the next 5 years is to inspire 20 million people around the globe to make a major change in their lives through better personal hygiene. Greg understands that hygiene is an often difficult topic for people to discuss but that doesn't hold him back in helping people. He aims to achieve this goal quickly, so he can move on to helping the next 20 million people to realize their higher purpose and fulfil their greatest potential in all areas of their life.

At the forefront of this quest is educating people about the personal, financial and environmental benefits of The Bum Gun bidet sprayer.

Free Books:

If you are interested in getting your hands on my FREE report titled:

"147 Ways To Improve Your Life That Everyone Should Know" please email me on: info@thebumgun.com

Please use the subject line "Send me my free copy of 147 Ways.." and I'll rush it over to you.

Discover Our Irresistible Offer:

Give The Bum Gun Bidet Sprayer a test run today. You Will NEVER regret it... That's a Promise!

www.thebumgun.com/irresistible-offer-a

One Last Thing

As you would have read in my author bio I have a plan to reach 20 million people around the globe with my **'5/20 Plan'** over the next 5 years. Of course this is a major plan and will help me make major changes in so many people's lives. And importantly to the environment so our future generations have a world with less problems than we face. To reach 20 million people at all **I need <u>your</u> help.**

If everyone who reads this report helps me connect with at least 5 of their friends, family and colleagues I have a real fighting chance of making this plan work. Therefore, I am asking you for help.

To be able to educate more people about the personal, financial and environmental benefits of The Bum Gun bidet sprayer I need you to do something for me.

Would you be able to send me the email addresses of 5 closest friends, family members and colleagues you think would be interested in reading this report? (greg@thebumgun.com)

Important Note: You have my complete word I will not spam them with junk or useless information. I will totally respect that these are special people in your life.

I only intend to share my free reports with them so that they too can discover the benefits of The Bum Gun.

Amazon Reviews

If you enjoyed reading this book and found it useful we would be very grateful if you would post a short review on Amazon. Your support **really does make a massive difference** and helps us reach more people to help improve their lives also. We read every single review personally so we can get your feedback to make The Bum Gun Series even better.

If you would like to leave a review, then all you need to do is click the review link on this book's page on Amazon.

Thank you again for all your awesome support.

Greg Noland

Connect with Greg Noland and The Bum Gun

For updates on The Bum Gun developments, follow us on **Twitter** at www.twitter.com/thebumgun

The Bum Gun Blog: www.thebumgun.com/the-bum-gun-blog/ for health and hygiene reports & tips, special offers, and funny news on health, hygiene and bathrooms in general ☺

Friend us on Facebook:

www.facebook.com/The.Bum.Gun.UK

If you are on **Instagram** – why not get in touch?

www.instagram.com/thebumgun/

"THE BUMGUN IS SIMPLE COMMON SENSE"

If anyone has a family, business or any commercial premises, they'd be wise to get this device of the century installed. Honestly, this is probably the best product I've purchased for a long time. It truly is a life changer. Hygiene is important for my family and my employees, and should be for you too.

The Bum Gun paid for itself in about 2 months. So you'd be crazy not to get one installed in every bathroom.

Thanks Bum Gun you really have an amazing product.

Hurz, Germany

Being Without The Bum Gun for 3 weeks was Absolute Torture

I recently spent 3 glorious weeks in Australia visiting friends. I must say the trip was absolutely fabulous from the moment i landed in Sydney. BUT, and this is a massive BUT, I missed my Bum Gun every day. For those of you who have already discovered the huge benefits of The Bum Gun you will know exactly what I mean. But I can well imagine those of you who are still using toilet paper will be wondering what the hell I am on about. Honestly though, being without The Bum Gun for 3 weeks was absolute torture. I had to make sure I was able to have a shower after every visit to the toilet, because I could just not bring myself to have to face the pain and uncleanliness of toilet paper.

You just have to take the plunge and get a bum gun installed in your bathroom for yourself to truly understand how massively better a jet of water is than toilet paper. Everyone can afford The Bum Gun so there is no excuse on price

The English Aussie

Excellent customer service and product

I found their products online and they are exactly what i needed. High quality all stainless steel, well-made and it has been working great since then. I highly recommend this store and products.

Fabrizio Morbini, Italy

Heavenly back crack DIY spray

After living in the land of smiles for a long while I one day ran out of paper and finally 'had a go'.

Yes I put my hand on the gun shaped spray device at the side of the toilet and had a squirt and a play.

It was a bit strange at first but it certainly did the job and the next day I was doing the reach around again for this neat clean little device.

What an invention! An amazing clean and feeling of freshness rather than running and smearing that brown bacteria filled mess back over your ass crack and thinking you're clean.

I can't understand why anyone in the UK once they have seen this device, and especially used one would ever go back to bog paper again!

It's refreshing and super clean and a satisfying feeling knowing that your ass is clean after your daily dump. Have a try you will see. Stay clean stay well stay fresh. I recommend this.

Jony Hirst, UK

"Here to a cleaner future, a great use around the toilet"

Just before Christmas I bought the Bum Gun bidet sprayer due to getting fed up of relying on my Biddy that was taking up room in what I already have a small bathroom but bigger than average. Now I have taken my Biday out I can now put in a washing basket and now worry about the hygiene of keeping clean. At first I was worried about any mess this would of caused but after using it, it was such a mess after all and fits in my bathroom with all the other bathroom wear without a notice. I also had my Bum Gun shower hose installed in under an hour which helped with any costs and if you're trying to decide if to buy one of these and have it fitted, I have no doubt in recommending the Bum Gun and you will feel the benefit immediately. Without sounding rude or anything, it has a great sensation feeling any dirty being cleaned away when using the Bum Gun well sat on the toilet. Even the plumber was amazed and now wants one.

Reyna, London, England

"Massive personal hygiene breakthrough"

"I was familiar already with the Asian style bidet sprayer and a convert from the start. When I came across the Bum Gun Company on returning to the UK I did not hesitate to order two sprayer kits, one for the bathroom and the other for the cloakroom toilet. They have been installed for nearly one month and are, predictably, a winner in every sense. Smart in appearance, adding style but above all comfortable and super hygienic to use while at the same time offering a massive saving on the use of toilet rolls, over time. This simple piece of kit is truly amazing but not as amazing as the timidity of the UK public to embrace the idea."

Frank Thomas, Gloucestershire, UK

"Save the planet without toilet paper"

My wife and I have just purchased the Mario model bidet sprayer from the Bum Gun. I wanted to write a review because of the excellent service I received but also because I am so happy at the quality of this bidet sprayer. I cannot believe I put up with toilet paper for so many years. This technology should have been invented by a German. For once our inventors have been outclassed, because this is an awesome upgrade from toilet paper. So much cleaner, more comfortable, and I am already noticing how much I am saving from my shopping bill now I don't have to buy so much toilet paper. Very impressed.

Nicholson, Germany

This help the feeling of well-being

Dear extended family, a clean behind is a feeling that cannot be described in details you simply have to experience it.

When you have started getting used to it you will suffer when you are out and have to adhere to the standard paper method.

So please, do yourself and your family a favour and get a simple version installed should you doubt it or go for a version where it is a permanent integrated part of the bathroom.

Personally we have installed it permanent in both our bathrooms and we cannot live without it as it gives you a superior feeling of well-being.

Chana, New Zealand

www.ingramcontent.com/pod-product-compliance
Lightning Source LLC
Chambersburg PA
CBHW060226290526
45789CB00003B/1428